Complete Air Fryer Cooking Guide

A Comprehensive Collection of Air Fryer Recipes from Breakfast to Dinner

By Samantha Hendrick

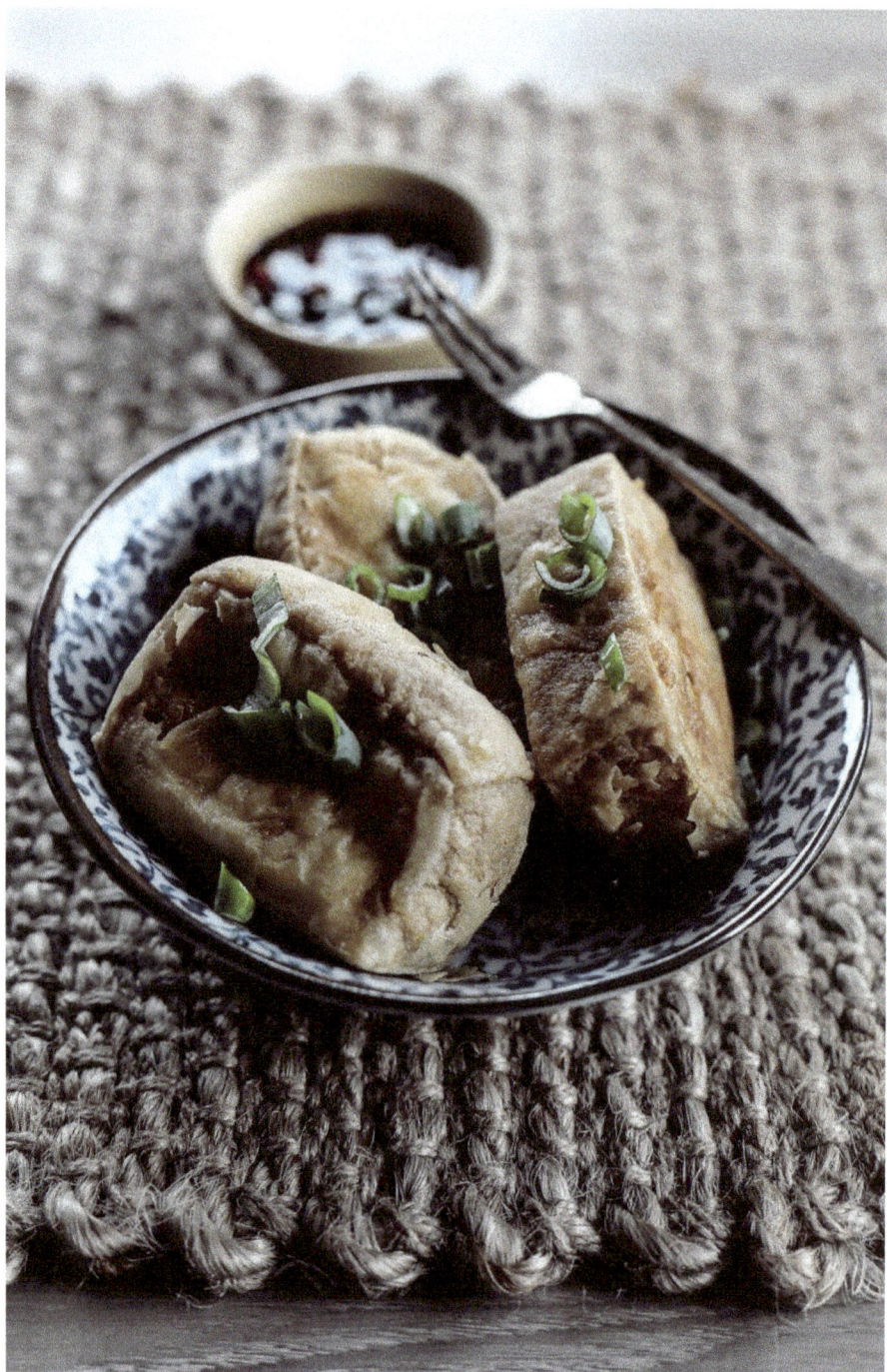

Table of Contents

Onion 'n Garlic Rubbed Trip Tip

Servings per Recipe: 4

Cooking Time: 50 minutes

Ingredients:

- ½ cup Burgandy or merlot wine vinegar /65ML
- 1 teaspoon garlic powder /5G
- 1 teaspoon onion powder /5G
- 1-pound beef tri-tip /450G
- 3 avocadoes, seeded and sliced
- 3 tablespoons essential olive oil /45ML

Instructions

1) Place all ingredients apart from the avocado slices in a Ziploc.
2) Place in a fridge allow to marinate for a couple of hours.
3) Preheat the air fryer to 3300F or 166°C .
4) Place the grill pan accessory in the air fryer.
5) Grill the avocado for just two minutes whilst the beef is marinating. Set aside.
6) After two hours, grill the beef for 50 minutes. Flip the beef halfway from the cooking time.
7) Serve the beef with grilled avocadoes

Nutrition information:

- Calories per serving: 515
- Carbs: 8g
- Protein: 33g
- Fat: 39g

Oregano-Paprika on Breaded Pork

Servings per Recipe: 4

Cooking Time: 30 minutes

Ingredients:

- ¼ cup water 62.5ML
- ¼ teaspoon dry mustard /1.25G
- ½ teaspoon black pepper /2.5G
- ½ teaspoon red pepper cayenne /2.5G
- ½ teaspoon garlic powder /2.5G
- ½ teaspoon salt /2.5G
- 1 cup panko breadcrumbs /130G
- 1 egg, beaten
- 2 teaspoons oregano /10G
- 4 lean pork chops
- 4 teaspoons paprika

Instructions:

1) Preheat the air fryer to 390°F or 199°C .
2) Use paper towels to pat dry the pork chops.
3) Add the egg and water. Then reserve.
4) In another bowl, combine the rest of the ingredients.
5) Dip the pork chops in the egg mixture and dredge within the flour mixture.

6) Place in mid-air fryer basket and cook for 25 to 30 minutes until golden.

Nutrition information:

- Calories per serving: 364
- Carbs: 2.5g
- Protein: 42.9g
- Fat: 20.2g

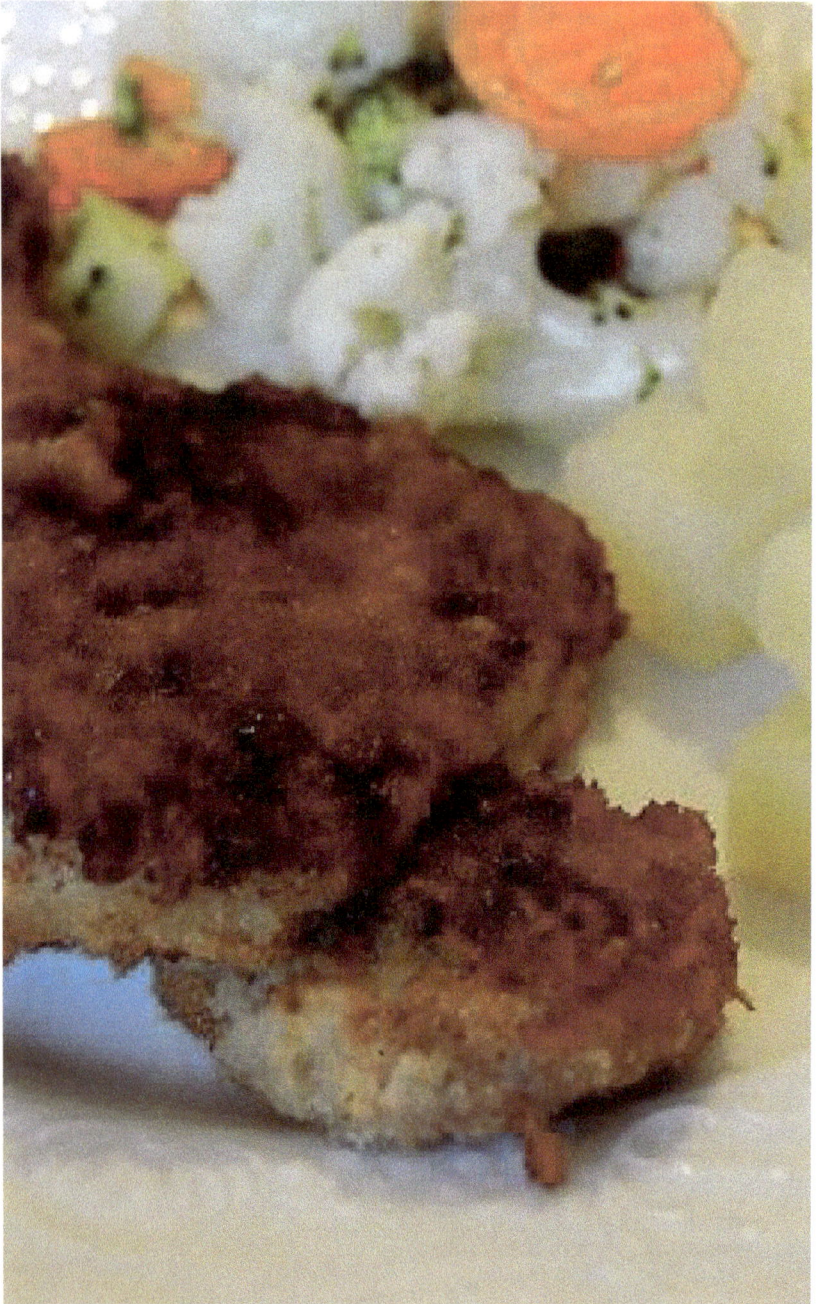

Paprika Beef 'n Bell Peppers Stir Fry

Servings per Recipe: 4

Cooking Time: 40 minutes

Ingredients:

- 1 ¼ pounds beef flank steak, sliced thinly /562.5G
- 1 red bell pepper, julienned
- 1 tablespoon red pepper cayenne /15G
- 1 tablespoon garlic powder /15G
- 1 tablespoon onion powder /15G
- 1 yellow bell pepper, julienned
- 3 tablespoons extra virgin olive oil /45ML
- 3 tablespoons paprika powder /45G
- Salt and pepper to taste

Instructions:

1) Preheat mid-air fryer to 390° F or 199°C .
2) Place the grill pan accessory in the air fryer.
3) Mix all ingredients in a bowl. Coat well.
4) Place this mix on the grill pan and cook for 40 minutes.
5) Make sure to stir every 10 minutes.

Nutrition information:

- Calories per serving: 334
- Carbs: 9.8g

- Protein: 32.5g
- Fat: 18.2g

Peach Puree on Ribeye

Servings per Recipe: 2

Cooking Time: 45 minutes

Ingredients:

- ¼ cup balsamic vinegar /62.5ML
- 1 cup peach puree /250ML
- 1 tablespoon paprika /15G
- 1 teaspoon thyme /5G
- 1-pound T-bone steak /450G
- 2 teaspoons lemon pepper seasoning /10G
- Salt and pepper to taste

Instructions:

1) Place all ingredients inside a Ziploc bag and allow to marinate in the fridge for around 120 minutes.
2) Preheat the air fryer to 390° F or 199°C .
3) Place the grill pan accessory in the air fryer.
4) Grill for 20 minutes and flip the meat halfway with the cooking time.

Nutrition information:

- Calories per serving: 570
- Carbs: 35.7g
- Protein: 47g

- Fat: 26.5g

Pickling 'n Jerk Spiced Pork

Servings per Recipe: 3

Cooking Time: 15 minutes

Ingredients:

- ½ cup ready-made jerk sauce /125ML
- 1 cup rum /250ML
- 1 cup water /250ML
- 1-lb pork tenderloin, sliced into 1-inch cubes /450G
- 2 teaspoons pickling spices /10G
- 3 tablespoons brown sugar /45G
- 3 tablespoons each salt /450G
- 4 garlic cloves

Instructions:

1) Boil water in a saucepan, allow to boil, add salt and brown sugar. Add garlic and pickling spices, stir and allow to simmer for 3 minutes. Remove from heat and stir in the rum.

2) Pour the sauce into a shallow dish. Add the pork tenderloin, stir and allow to marinate in the refrigerator for 3 hours.

3) Skewer the pork pieces. Baste with the marinade. Place the skewer on the skewer rack in the air fryer.

4) Cook at 360° F or 183°C for 12 minutes. Turnover skewers and baste with sauce after 6 minutes. If need be, cook in batches.

5) Serve and enjoy.

Nutrition Information:

- Calories per Serving: 295
- Carbs: 19.9g
- Protein: 41.0g
- Fat: 5.7g

Crispy Lemon-Parsley Fish Cakes

Serves: 3

Cooking Time: 20 minutes

Ingredients:

- ½ cup dried coconut flakes /65g
- 1 cup almond flour /130g
- 1 cup cooked salmon, shredded /130g
- 1 tablespoon chopped parsley /15g
- 1 tablespoon freshly squeezed lemon juice /15ml
- 2 eggs, beaten
- 3 tablespoons coconut oil /45ml
- Salt and pepper to taste

Instructions:

1) Combine the salmon, almond flour, eggs, salt, pepper, fresh lemon juice and parsley in a large bowl. Form a thick dough.
2) Form small round balls with your hands and coat them in coconut flakes.
3) Brush the balls with coconut oil.
4) Preheat air fryer at 3250 F or 163°C .
5) Place the balls in a mid-air fryer basket and cook for 20 Minutes.

6) Shake the basket after 10 minutes of cooking.

Nutrition information:

- Calories per serving: 490
- Carbohydrates: 9.9g
- Protein: 35.5g
- Fat: 34.2g

Crispy Shrimps the Cajun Way

Serves: 3

Cooking Time: 8 minutes

Ingredients:

- ¼ teaspoon red pepper cayenne /1.25g
- ¼ teaspoon smoked paprika /1.25g
- ½ pound tiger shrimps /2.5g
- ½ teaspoon old bay seasoning /2.5g
- 3 tablespoons olive oil /45ml
- A pinch of salt

Instructions:

1) Put on your air fryer and warm for 5 minutes.
2) Mix all ingredients in a bowl and then place the bowl in an air fryer.
3) Place the shrimps in a mid-air fryer basket and cook for 8 minutes at 3900 F or 199°C .

Nutrition information:

- Calories per serving: 213
- Carbohydrates: 0.3g
- Protein: 15.4g
- Fat: 16.7g

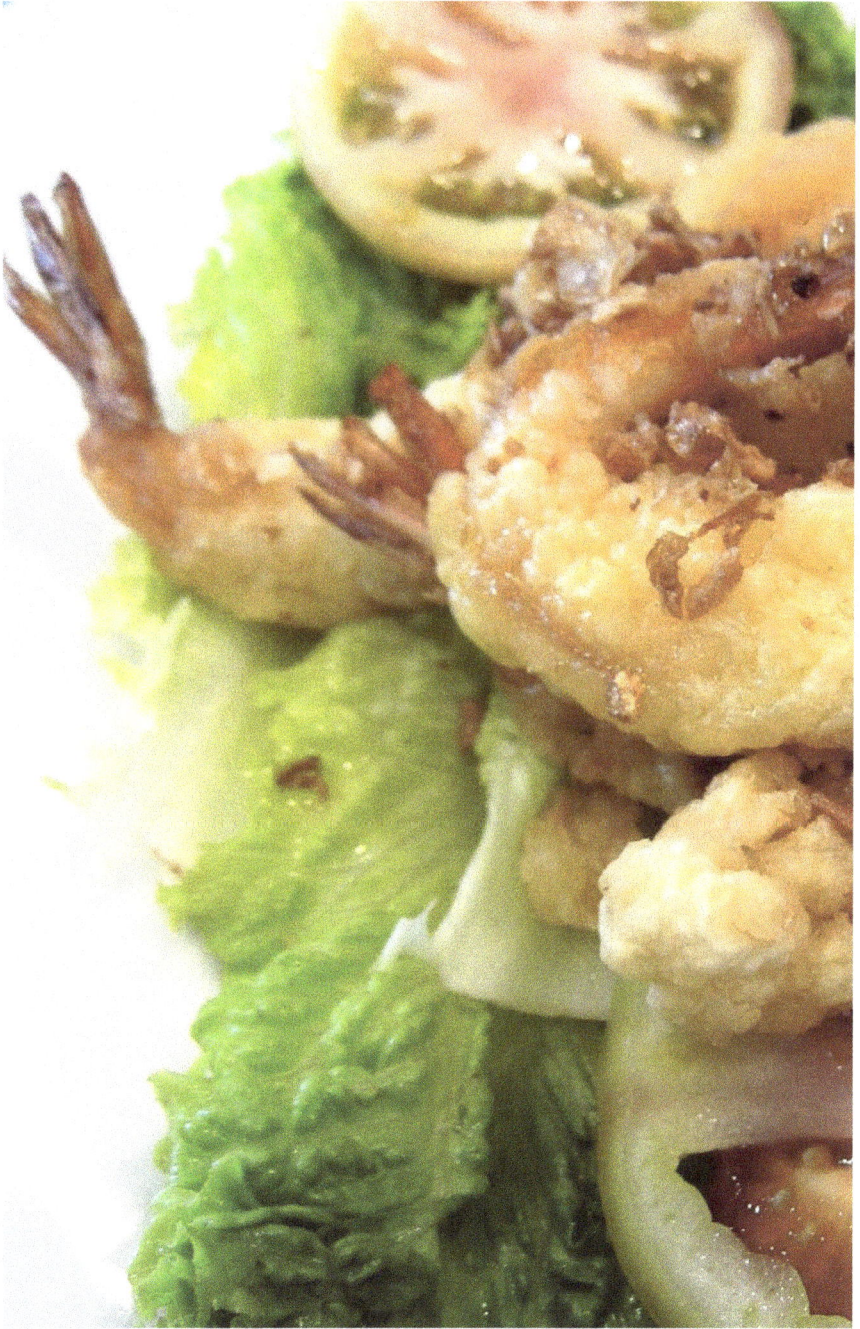

Crispy Spicy-Lime Fish Filet

Serves: 4

Cooking Time: 15

Ingredients:

- 1 egg white, beaten
- 1 tablespoon lime juice, freshly squeezed /15ml
- 1 teaspoon lime zest /5g
- 2 fish fillets, cut into pieces
- 2 tablespoons extra virgin olive oil /30ml
- 5 tablespoons almond flour /75g
- A dash of chili powder
- Salt and pepper to taste

Instructions:

1) Warm-up mid-air fryer for 5 minutes.
2) Place all ingredients in a Ziploc bag and shake until all ingredients are very well combined.
3) Place in the air fryer basket.
4) Cook for 15 minutes at 4000 F or 205°C .

Nutrition information:

- Calories per serving: 192
- Carbohydrates: 9.63g
- Protein: 8.14g

- Fat: 13.14g

Cumin, Thyme 'n Oregano Herbed Shrimps

Servings per Recipe: 4

Cooking Time: 6 minutes

Ingredients:

- ¼ teaspoon red pepper cayenne /1.25g
- ¼ teaspoon red chili flakes /1.25g
- 1 teaspoon cumin /5g
- 1 teaspoon oregano /5g
- 1 teaspoon salt /5g
- 1 teaspoon thyme /5g
- 2 tablespoons coconut oil /30g
- 2 teaspoons cilantro /10g
- 2 teaspoons onion powder /10g
- 2 teaspoons smoked paprika /10g
- 20 jumbo shrimps, peeled and deveined

Instructions:

1) Preheat the air fryer to 3900 F or 199°C .
2) Season the shrimps with the Ingredients.
3) Place the seasoned shrimps within the double layer rack.
4) Cook for 6 minutes.

Nutrition information:

- Calories per serving: 220
- Carbs: 2.5g
- Protein: 34.2g
- Fat: 8.1g

Crispy and Spicy Hot Shrimps

Serves: 6

Cooking Time: 5 minutes

Ingredients:

- ½ teaspoon ground black pepper /2.5g
- ½ teaspoon salt /2.5g
- 1 teaspoon chili flakes /5g
- 1 teaspoon chili powder /5g
- 12 fresh prawns, peeled and deveined
- 4 tablespoons essential olive oil /60ml

Instructions:

1) Warm up the air fryer for 5 minutes.
2) Find a bowl that can fit in your air fryer and mix all ingredients in it.
3) Place the shrimps in the air fryer basket and cook for 5 minutes at 4000 F or 205°C .

Nutrition information:

- Calories per serving: 156
- Carbohydrates: 0.8g
- Protein: 15.3g
- Fat: 10.2g

Spiced Coco-Lime Skewered Shrimp

Servings per Recipe: 6

Cooking Time: 12 minutes

Ingredients:

- 1 lime, zested and juiced
- 1/3 cup chopped fresh cilantro /43G
- 1/3 cup shredded coconut /43G
- 1/4 cup essential olive oil /62.5ML
- 1/4 cup soy sauce /62.5ML
- 1-pound uncooked medium shrimp, peeled and deveined /450G
- 2 garlic cloves
- 2 jalapeno peppers, seeded

Instructions:

1) Blend the soy sauce, extra virgin olive oil, coconut oil, cilantro, garlic, lime juice, lime zest, and jalapeno until smooth.
2) Mix shrimp and processed marinade in a bowl. Stir well to coat. Place in a fridge to marinate for 3 hours.
3) Thread shrimps in skewers. Place on skewer rack in the air fryer.
4) At 360° F or 183°C cook for 6 minutes. Cook in batches if required.

5) Serve and enjoy while eating.

Nutrition Information:

- Calories per Serving: 172
- Carbs: 4.8g
- Protein: 13.4g
- Fat: 10.9g

Sweet Honey-Hoisin Glazed Salmon

Servings per Recipe: 2

Cooking Time: 12 minutes

Ingredients:

- 1 tablespoon honey /15ML
- 1 tablespoon olive oil /15ML
- 1 tablespoon rice wine /15ML
- 1 tablespoon soy sauce /15ML
- 1-lb salmon filet, cut into 2-inch rectangles /450G
- 3 tablespoons hoisin sauce /45ML

Instructions:

1) Add all ingredients to a shallow bowl and mix properly. Allow to marinate in the refrigerator for 3 hours.
2) Thread salmon pieces in skewers and reserve marinade for sprinkling. Place on skewer rack in the air fryer.
3) At 360° F or 183°C cook for 12 minutes. Halfway through cooking time, turnover skewers and baste with marinade. If needed, cook in batches.
4) Serve and enjoy.

Nutrition Information:

- Calories per Serving: 971
- Carbs: 23.0g

- Protein: 139.4g
- Fat: 35.7g

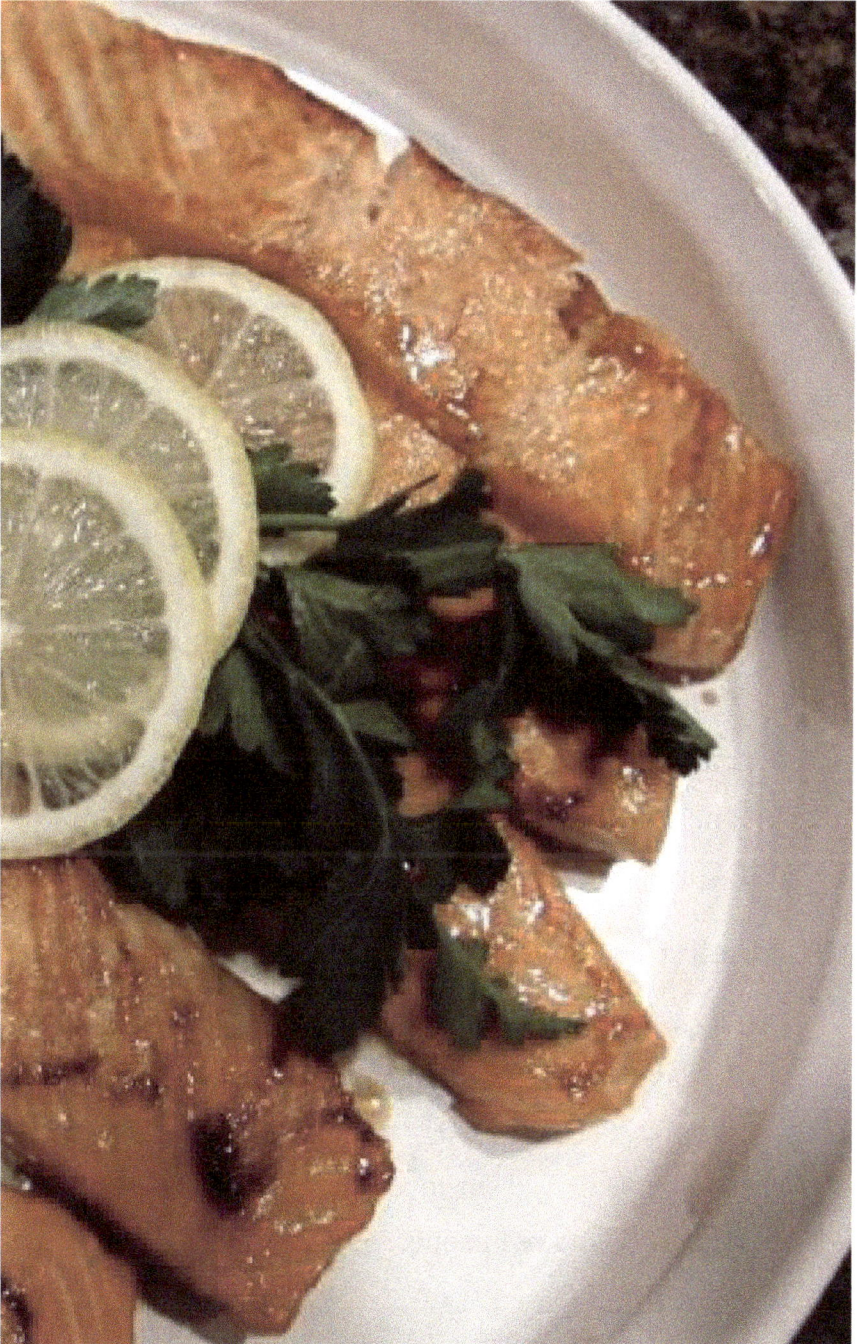

Sweet-Chili Sauce Dip 'n Shrimp Rolls

Servings per Recipe: 8

Cooking Time: 9 minutes

Ingredients:

- ¼ teaspoon crushed red pepper /1.25G
- ½ cup sweet chili sauce /125ML
- ¾ cup snow peas, julienned /88G
- 1 cup carrots, julienned /130G
- 1 cup red bell pepper, seeded and julienned /130G
- 2 ½ tablespoons sesame oil, divided /38ML
- 2 cups cabbage, shredded /260G
- 2 teaspoons fish sauce /10ML
- 4 ounces raw shrimps, deveined and chopped /120G
- 8 spring roll wrappers

Instructions:

1) Place a saucepan over medium heat. Add sesame oil, add the cabbage, carrots, and bell pepper and stir for just two minutes. Set aside.
2) Once cooled, Add shrimps and snow peas. Season with fish sauce and red pepper.

3) Place the spring roll wrapper on a flat surface and put a tablespoon or two of the vegetable mixtures in the middle. Wrap the spring roll wrapper and seal the edges with water.

4) Preheat the air fryer to 390° F or 199°C .

5) Place the spring rolls in the double layer rack. Spray with olive oil.

6) Cook for 7 minutes.

7) Serve with chili sauce.

Nutrition information:

- Calories per serving: 185
- Carbs: 19g
- Protein: 7g
- Fat: 9g

Tartar Sauce 'n Crispy Cod Nuggets

Servings per Recipe: 3

Cooking Time: 10 Minutes

Ingredients:

- ½ cup flour /65G
- ½ cup non-fat mayonnaise /125ML
- ½ teaspoon Worcestershire sauce /2.5ML
- 1 ½ pounds cod fillet /675G
- 1 cup cracker crumbs /130G
- 1 egg, beaten
- 1 tablespoon sweet pickle relish /15G
- 1 tablespoon vegetable oil /15ML
- 1 teaspoon honey /5ML
- Juice from half a lemon
- Salt and pepper to taste
- Zest from half of a lemon

Instructions:

1) Preheat mid-air fryer to 390° F or 199°C .
2) Season the cod fillets with salt and pepper to taste.
3) Dip the fish in the flour, then in the beaten egg and then coat with the cracker crumbs. Brush all sides with oil.
4) Place the fish on the double layer rack and cook for 10 minutes.

5) Meanwhile, prepare the sauce by mixing all ingredients in a bowl.

6) Serve the fish using the sauce.

Nutrition information:

- Calories per serving: 470
- Carbs: 25.4g
- Protein: 42.9g
- Fat: 21.8g

Tomato 'n Onion Stuffed Grilled Squid

Servings per Recipe: 4

Cooking Time: 15

Ingredients:

- ½ cup green onions, chopped /65G
- ½ cup tomatoes, chopped /65G
- 1 tablespoon fresh lemon juice /15ML
- 2 pounds squid, gutted and cleaned /900G
- 2 tablespoons organic olive oil /30ML
- 5 cloves of garlic
- Salt and pepper to taste

Instructions:

1) Preheat mid-air fryer to 390° F or 199°C .
2) Place the grill pan in the air fryer.
3) Season the squid with salt, pepper, and freshly squeezed lemon juice.
4) Stuff the hollow with garlic, tomatoes, and onions.
5) Brush the squid with essential olive oil.
6) Place on the grill pan and cook for 15 minutes.
7) Halfway through the cooking time, flip the squid.

Nutrition information:

- Calories per serving: 277

- Carbs: 10.7g
- Protein: 36g
- Fat: 10g

Fried Broccoli Recipe From India

Serves: 6

Cooking Time: 15

Ingredients

- ¼ teaspoon turmeric powder /1.25G
- ½ pounds broccoli, cut into florets /2.5G
- 1 tablespoon almond flour /15G
- 1 teaspoon garam masala /5G
- 2 tablespoons coconut milk /30ML
- ·Salt and pepper to taste

Instructions:

1) Preheat the air fryer for 5 minutes.
2) Mix all ingredients in a bowl. Coat the broccoli florets with the other ingredients.
3) Place the broccoli florets in an air fryer basket and cook for 15 minutes until crispy.

Nutrition information:

- Calories per serving: 96
- Carbohydrates: 8.9g
- Protein: 3.1g
- Fat: 6.9g

Fried Chickpea-Fig on Arugula

Serves: 4

Cooking Time: 20 minutes

Ingredients

- 1 ½ cups chickpeas, cooked /195G
- 1 teaspoon cumin seeds, roasted then crushed /5G
- 2 tablespoons extra-virgin essential olive oil /30ML
- 3 cups arugula rocket, washed and dried /390G
- 4 tablespoons balsamic vinegar /60ML
- 8 fresh figs, halved
- salt and pepper to taste

Instructions

1) Preheat air fryer to 375° F or 191°C .
2) Line the air fryer basket with aluminium foil and brush with oil.
3) Place the figs inside the air fryer and cook for 10 minutes.
4) Mix the chickpeas and cumin seeds in a bowl properly.
5) Cook the chickpeas for 10 minutes. Allow to cool
6) Combine the balsamic vinegar, organic olive oil, salt and pepper in a bowl and mix well.
7) Place the arugula rocket in a salad bowl and add the cooled figs and chickpeas.

8) Pour the sauce over the content of the salad bowl and mix to coat.

9) Serve immediately.

Nutrition information:

- Calories per serving: 388
- Carbohydrates: 62.51g
- Protein:16.72 g
- Fat:7.92 g

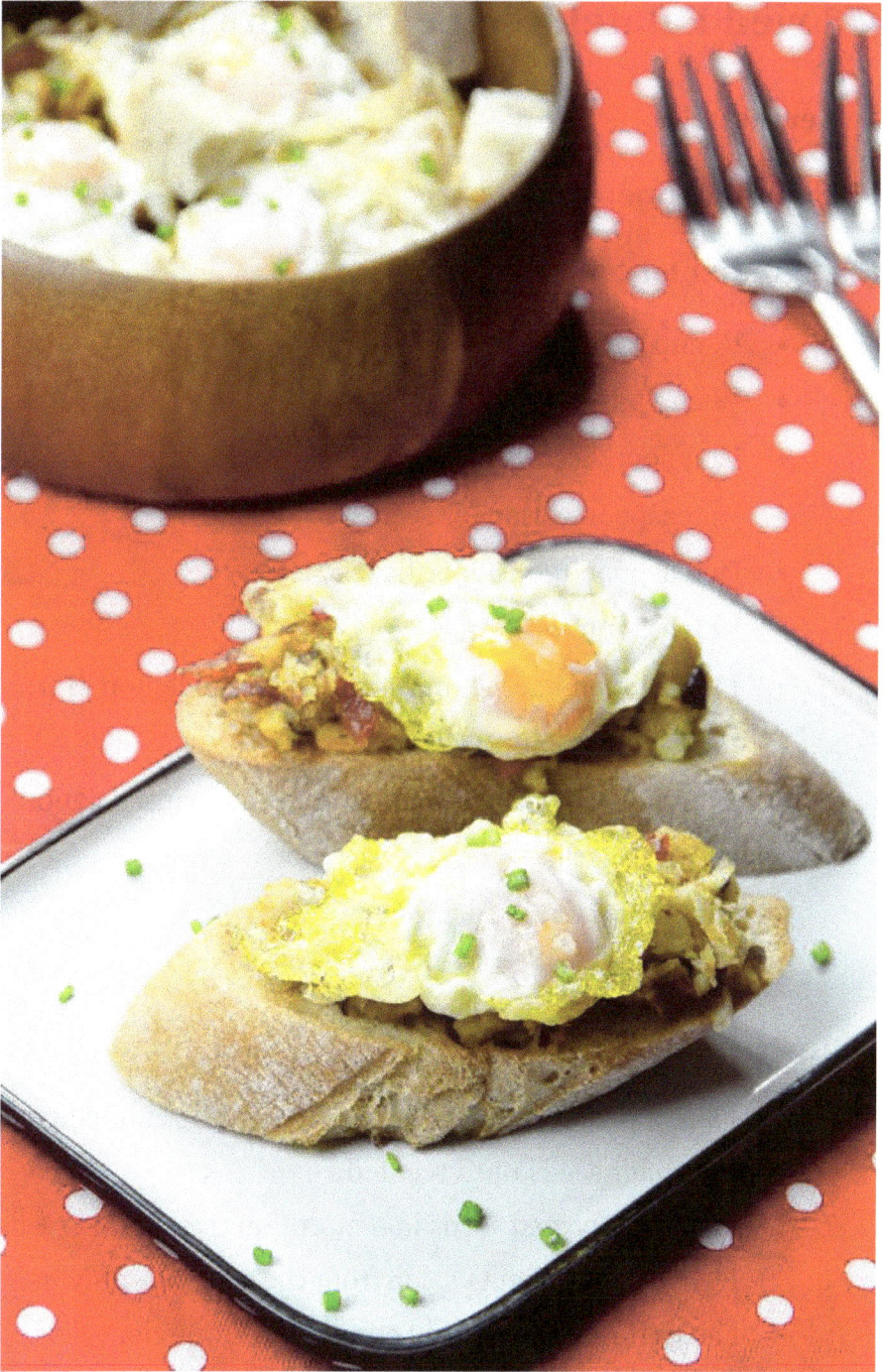

Fried Falafel Recipe from the Middle East

Serves: 8

Cooking Time: 15

Ingredients:

- ¼ cup coriander, chopped /32.5G
- ¼ cup parsley, chopped /32.5G
- ½ onion, diced
- ½ teaspoon coriander seeds /2.5G
- ½ teaspoon red pepper flakes /2.5G
- ½ teaspoon salt /2.5G
- 1 tablespoon juice from freshly squeezed lemon /15ML
- 1 teaspoon cumin seeds /5G
- 2 cups chickpeas from can, drained and rinsed /260G
- ·3 cloves garlic
- 3 tablespoons all-purpose flour /45G
- cooking spray

Instructions:

1) Place a pan over a medium heat, toast the cumin and coriander seeds until scented.
2) Place the toasted seeds in a mortar and crush the seeds.
3) Place all ingredients aside from the cooking spray in a blender. Add the toasted cumin and coriander seeds.
4) Blend until fine.

5) Shape the amalgamation into falafels and spray olive oil.

6) Place within a preheated air fryer and make sure that they don't overlap.

7) Cook at 400° F or 205°C for 15 minutes or until the surface becomes golden brown.

Nutrition information:

- Calories per serving: 110
- Carbohydrates: 18.48g
- Protein: 5.11g
- Fat: 1.72g

Fried Tofu Recipe from Malaysia

Servings per Recipe: 4

Cooking Time: 30 Minutes

Ingredients:

- 1 block tofu, cut into strips
- 1 tablespoon maple syrup /15ML
- 1 teaspoon sriracha sauce /5ML
- 2 cloves of garlic
- 2 tablespoons soy sauce /30ML
- 2 teaspoons fresh ginger no need to peel, coarsely chopped /10G
- juice of just one fresh lime

- Peanut Butter Sauce Ingredients

- 1 tablespoon soy sauce /15ML
- 1/2 cup creamy peanut butter /65G
- 1-2 teaspoons Sriracha sauce to taste /10ML
- 2 cloves of garlic
- 2-inch little bit of fresh ginger coarsely chopped
- 6 tablespoons of water /90ML
- juice of merely one/2 a fresh lemon

Instructions:

1) Blend all peanut butter sauce ingredients until smooth and creamy. Transfer into a medium bowl and place aside for dipping sauce.
2) Blend garlic, sriracha, ginger, maple syrup, lime juice, and soy sauce until smooth. Pour into a bowl and add strips of tofu, Marinate for 30 minutes.
3) Skewer tofu strips.
4) Place on skewer rack and air fry for 15 at 370° F or 188°C .
5) Serve and enjoy.

Nutrition Information:

- Calories per Serving: 347
- Carbs: 16.6g
- Protein: 16.6g
- Fat: 23.8g

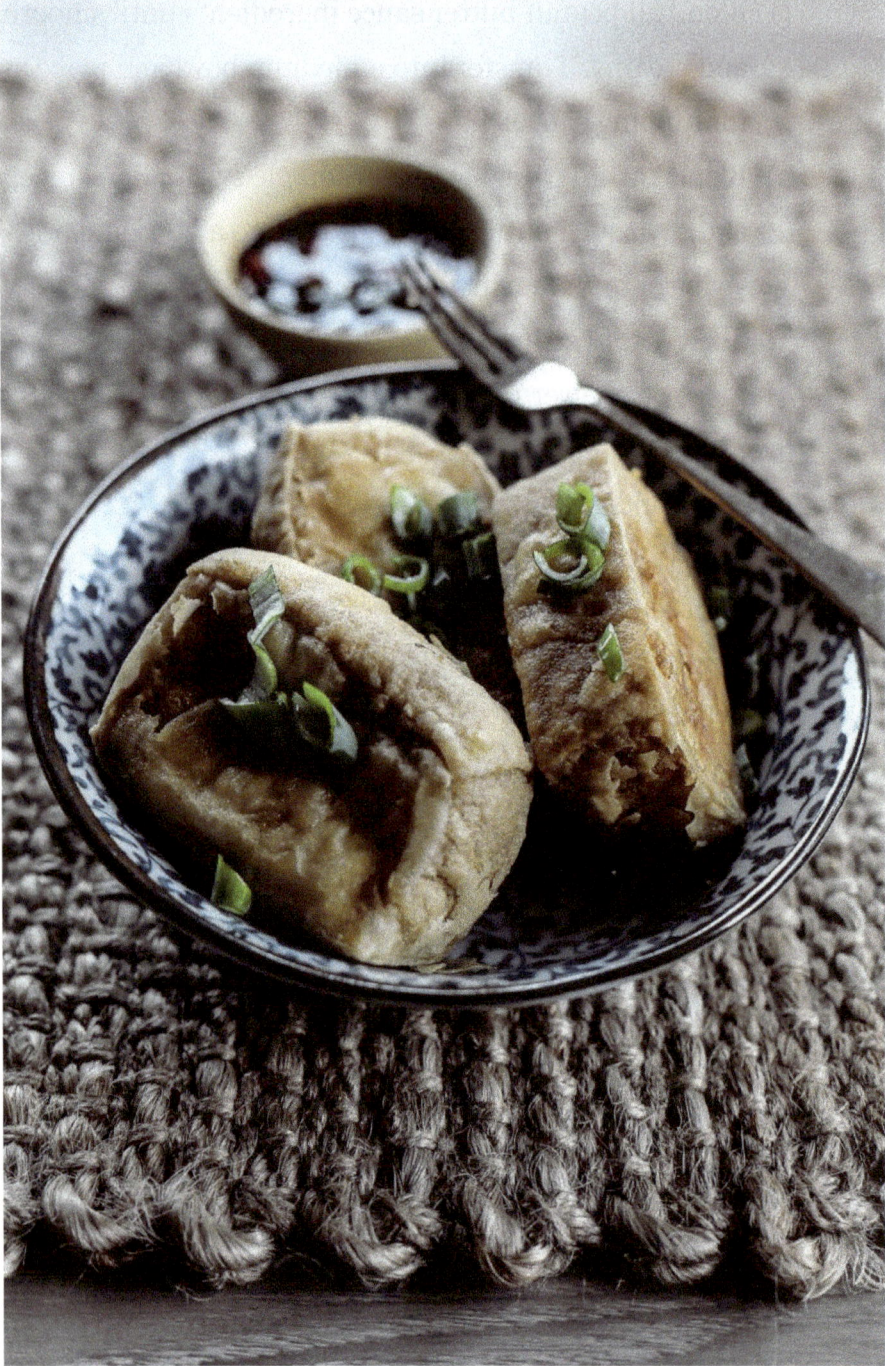

Garlic 'n Basil Crackers

Serves: 6

Cooking Time: 15 minutes

Ingredients:

- ¼ teaspoon dried basil powder /1.25G
- ½ teaspoon baking powder /2.5G
- 1 ¼ cups almond flour /162.5G
- 1 clove of garlic, minced
- 3 tablespoons coconut oil /45ML
- A pinch of red pepper cayenne powder
- Salt and pepper to taste

Instructions:

1) Preheat the air fryer for 5 minutes.
2) Mix everything in a mixing bowl to make a dough.
3) Transfer the dough to a clean and flat surface and knead until 2mm thick. Cut into squares.
4) Place gently in mid-air fryer basket. Do this in batches if you like.
5) Cook for 15 minutes at 325° F or 163°C .

Nutrition information:

- Calories per serving: 206
- Carbohydrates: 2.9g

- Protein: 5.3g
- Fat: 19.3g

Sweet 'n Nutty Marinated Cauliflower-Tofu

Serves: 2

Cooking Time: 20 minutes

Ingredients:

- ¼ cup brown sugar /32.5G
- ¼ cup low sodium soy sauce /62.5ML
- ½ teaspoon chili garlic sauce /125ML
- 1 package extra-firm tofu, pressed to produce extra water and cut into cubes
- 1 small head cauliflower, cut into florets
- 1 tablespoon sesame oil /15ML
- 2 ½ tablespoons almond butter /37.5G
- 2 cloves of garlic, minced

Instructions:

1) Whisk properly the garlic, sesame oil, soy sauce, sugar, chili garlic sauce, and almond butter together in a mixing bowl;
2) Place the tofu cubes and cauliflower in the mix. Allow to take up the sauce for 30 minutes.
3) Preheat the air fryer to 400° F or 205°C . Add tofu and cauliflower. Cook for 20 Minutes. Flip the air fryer basket halfway through the cooking time.

4) Put the remaining marinade in the saucepan and place safe it on medium heat. Once it starts boiling reduce the heat to low, and stir utensil sauce thickens.

5) Pour the sauce within the tofu and cauliflower.

6) Serve with rice or noodles.

Nutrition information:

- Calories per serving: 365
- Carbohydrates: 40.1g
- Protein: 9.85g
- Fat: 18.38g

Tender Butternut Squash Fry

Servings per Recipe: 2

Cooking Time: 10 minutes

Ingredients:

- 1 tablespoon cooking oil /15ML
- 1-pound butternut squash, seeded and sliced /450G
- Salt and pepper to taste

Instructions

1) Place the grill pan in the mid-air fryer.
2) Place all ingredients in a bowl, mix and season the squash.
3) Place in the grill pan.
4) Close the air fryer and cook for 10 minutes at 330° F or 166°C .

Nutrition information:

- Calories per serving: 171
- Carbs: 28.6g
- Protein: 2.7g
- Fat: 7.1g

Tofu Bites Soaked in Chili-Ginger Peanut Butter

Serves: 3

Cooking Time: 15 minutes

Ingredients:

- ¼ cup liquid aminos /62.5ML
- ¼ cup maple syrup /62.5ML
- 1 block extra firm tofu, pressed to remove excess water and cut into cubes
- 1 sprig cilantro, chopped
- 1 teaspoon red pepper flakes /5G
- 1 teaspoon sesame seeds /5G
- 1-inch fresh ginger, peeled and grated
- 2 cloves of garlic, minced
- 2 tablespoons rice wine vinegar /30ML
- 2 tablespoons sesame oil /30ML
- 3 tablespoon chili garlic sauce /45ML
- 3 tablespoons peanut butter /45G
- toasted peanuts, chopped

Instructions:

1) Place the first 9 ingredients in a bowl, mix well and pour in a Ziploc bag, add the tofu cubes. Allow to marinate for half an hour.

2) Preheat air fryer to 425° F or 219°C .

3) Save the marinade for later. Place the marinated tofu cubes in the mid-air fryer and cook for 15 minutes.

4) Pour the marinade in a saucepan and heat over medium flame until reduced by 50%.

5) Place the cooked tofu on top of the steaming rice and pour n the sauce. Garnish with toasted peanuts, sesame seeds and cilantro.

Nutrition information:

- Calories per serving: 484
- Carbohydrates: 32.42g
- Protein: 20.11g
- Fat: 30.43g

Twice-Fried Cauliflower Tater Tots

Serves: 12

Cooking Time: 16 minutes

Ingredients:

- ½ cup bread crumbs /65G
- ½ cup nutritional yeast /65G
- 1 flax egg (1 tablespoon 3 tablespoon desiccated coconuts) /15G+45G
- 1 onion, chopped
- 1 teaspoon chives, chopped /5G
- 1 teaspoon garlic, minced /5G
- 1 teaspoon oregano, chopped /5G
- 1 teaspoon parsley, chopped /5G
- 1-pound cauliflower, steamed and chopped /450G
- 3 tablespoons oats /45G
- flaxseed meal + 3 tablespoon water) /45ml
- salt and pepper to taste

Instructions:

1) Preheat the air fryer to 390 ° F or 199°C .
2) Place the steamed cauliflower on a paper towel and squeeze to get rid of excess water.
3) Place inside a mixing bowl and add other ingredients except for the bread crumbs.

4) Mix until well combined and form balls with your hands.

5) Roll the tater tots in the bread crumbs, ensuring it coats every part of the tater tots and place them in an air fryer.

6) Cook for 6 minutes. Once done, increase the cooking temperature to 400° F or 205°C and cook for another 10 minutes.

Nutrition information:

- Calories per serving: 47
- Carbohydrates: 7.54g
- Protein: 4.19g
- Fat: 0.52g

Chili-Espresso Marinated Steak

Servings per Recipe: 3

Cooking Time: 50 minutes

Ingredients:

- ½ teaspoon garlic powder /2.5G
- 1 ½ pounds beef flank steak /675G
- 1 teaspoon instant espresso powder /5G
- 2 tablespoons olive oil /30ML
- 2 teaspoons chili powder /10G
- Salt and pepper to taste

Instructions:

1) Preheat the air fryer to 390° F or 199°C .
2) Place the grill pan in the air fryer.
3) Mix the chili powder, salt, pepper, espresso powder, and garlic powder in a bowl.
4) Lavishly rub the seasoning on the steak and brush with oil.
5) Place on the grill pan and cook for 40 minutes.
6) Halfway from the cooking time, flip the beef to cook evenly.

Nutrition information:

- Calories per serving: 249

- Carbs: 4g
- Protein: 20g
- Fat: 17g

Chives on Bacon & Cheese Bake

Servings per Recipe: 6

Cooking Time: 50 minutes

Ingredients:

- 4 slices bread, crusts removed
- 1 cup egg substitute (for example Egg Beaters®) /250ML
- 1 tablespoon chopped fresh chives /15G
- 6 slices cooked bacon, crumbled
- 1 cup Cheddar cheese /130G
- 1 1/2 cups skim milk /375G

Instructions:

1) Cook bacon in a baking pan of air fryer for 10 minutes at 360° F or 183°C . Once done, remove excess fat then crush bacon.
2) Whisk eggs, stir in milk and chives.
3) In the same air fryer baking pan, evenly spread bread slices. Pour the egg mixture over it. Top with bacon. Cover the pan with foil and let it sit in the fridge for not less than 1 hour.
4) Preheat air fryer to 330° F or 166°C .
5) Cook while covered in foil for 20 Minutes. Remove foil and sprinkle cheese. Continue cooking uncovered for an additional 15 minutes.

6) Serve and enjoy

Nutrition Information:

- Calories per Serving: 207
- Carbs: 12.1g
- Protein: 15.3g
- Fat: 10.8g

Cilantro-Mint Pork BBQ Thai Style

Servings per Recipe: 3

Cooking Time: 15 minutes

Ingredients:

- 1 minced hot chile
- 1 minced shallot
- 1-pound ground pork /450G
- 2 tablespoons fish sauce /30ML
- 2 tablespoons lime juice /30ML
- 3 tablespoons basil /45G
- 3 tablespoons chopped mint /45G
- 3 tablespoons cilantro /45G

Instructions:

1) Place all ingredients in a shallow dish, using your hands mix properly and make 1-inch balls.
2) Skewer the balls and place them on the skewer rack in the air fryer.
3) For 15 minutes, cook on 360° F or 183°C . Halfway through cooking time, turnover skewers. If needed, cook in batches.
4) Serve and enjoy

Nutrition Information:

- Calories per Serving: 455
- Carbs: 2.5g
- Protein: 40.2g
- Fat: 31.5g

Coriander Lamb with Pesto 'n Mint Dip

Servings per Recipe: 4

Cooking Time: 16 minutes

Ingredients:

- 1 1/2 teaspoons coriander seeds, ground in a spice mill or perhaps mortar with pestle /7.5G
- 1 large red bell pepper, cut into 1-inch squares
- 1 small red onion, cut into 1-inch squares
- 1 tablespoon extra-virgin extra virgin olive oil plus additional for brushing /15ML
- 1 teaspoon coarse kosher salt /5G
- 1-pound trimmed lamb meat, cut into 1 1/4-inch cube /450G
- 4 large garlic cloves, minced

Mint-Pesto Dip Ingredients:

- 1 cup (packed) fresh mint leaves /130G
- 2 tablespoons pine nuts /30G
- 2 tablespoons freshly grated Parmesan cheese /30G
- 1 tablespoon fresh lemon juice /15ML
- 1 medium garlic herb, peeled
- 1/2 cup (packed) fresh cilantro leaves /65G
- 1/2 teaspoon coarse kosher salt /2.5G
- 1/2 cup (or even more) extra-virgin olive oil /65ML

Instructions:

1) In a blender, puree all Mint-Pesto dip Ingredients until smooth and creamy. Transfer to a bowl and set aside.

2) Mix coriander, salt, garlic, and oil in a large bowl. Add lamb, mix well to coat. Place in a fridge and allow to marinate for no less than 1 hour.

3) Thread lamb, bell pepper, and onion alternately in a skewer. Repeat until all ingredients are used. Place in skewer rack in the air fryer.

4) For 8 minutes, cook at 390° F or 199°C . Halfway through cooking time, turnover.

5) Serve and dress with sauce.

Nutrition Information:

- Calories per Serving: 307
- Carbs: 6.3g
- Protein: 21.1g
- Fat: 21.9

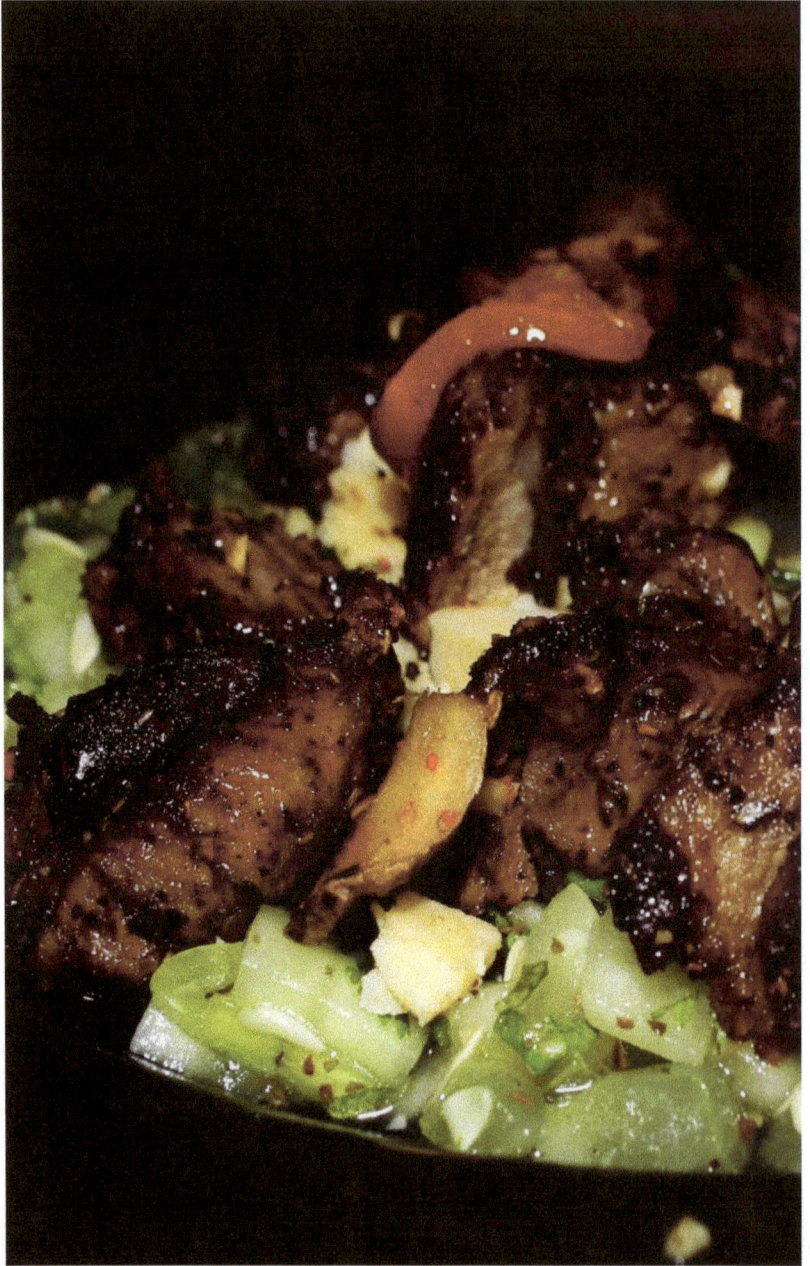

Coriander, Mustard 'n Cumin Rubbed Flank Steak

Servings per Recipe: 3

Cooking Time: 45 minutes

Ingredients:

- ½ teaspoon coriander /2.5G
- ½ teaspoon ground cumin /2.5G
- 1 ½ pounds flank steak /675G
- 1 tablespoon chili powder /15G
- 1 tablespoon paprika /15G
- 1 teaspoon garlic powder /5G
- 1 teaspoon mustard powder /5G
- 2 tablespoons sugar /30G
- 2 teaspoons black pepper /10G
- 2 teaspoons salt /10G

Instructions:

1) Preheat the air fryer to 390° F or 199°C .
2) Place the grill pan in the mid-air fryer.
3) Add all the spices into a small bowl and rub lavishly on the steak.
4) Place in the grill and cook for 15 minutes per batch.
5) Turn over the meat every 8 minutes for even grilling.

Nutrition information:

- Calories per serving: 330
- Carbs: 10.2g
- Protein:50 g
- Fat:12.1 g

Tri-Tip in Agave Nectar & Red Wine Marinade

Servings per Recipe: 4

Cooking Time: 40 minutes

Ingredients:

- ¼ cup dark wine /62.5ML
- 1 tablespoon agave nectar /15ML
- 1 tablespoon smoked paprika /15G
- 2 cloves of garlic, minced
- 2 cups chopped parsley /260G
- 2 pounds tri-tip steak, pounded /900G
- 2 tablespoons extra virgin olive oil /30ML
- Salt and pepper to taste

Instructions:

1) Place all ingredients in a Ziploc bag and allow it to marinate for about an hour.
2) Preheat air fryer to 390° F or 199°C .
3) Place the grill pan accessory in the air fryer.
4) Grill the meat for 40 minutes, turn it over frequently for even cooking

Nutrition information:

- Calories per serving: 667

- Carbs: 4.4g
- Protein: 69.3g
- Fat: 41.3g

Tri-Tip Skewers Hungarian Style

Servings per Recipe: 3

Cooking Time: 12 minutes

Ingredients:

- 1-lb beef tri-tip, sliced to 2-inch cubes /450G
- 2 smashed garlic cloves
- a pinch of salt
- 2 teaspoons crushed caraway seeds /10G
- 1 medium red onion, sliced into quarters
- 1 medium bell pepper seeded and cut into chunks
- 1/2 cup organic olive oil /125ML
- 1/2 teaspoon paprika /2.5G

Instructions:

1) Place all ingredients aside from bell pepper and onion in a bowl. Mix well to coat. Allow to marinate in the fridge for 3 hours.
2) Skewer beef, onion, and bell pepper. Place on skewer rack in the air fryer.
3) Cook at 360° F or 183°C for 6 minutes, turnover skewers and cook for another 6 minutes. If needed, cook in batches.
4) Serve, eat and enjoy.

Nutrition Information:

- Calories per Serving: 530
- Carbs: 3.3g
- Protein: 33.1g
- Fat: 42.7g

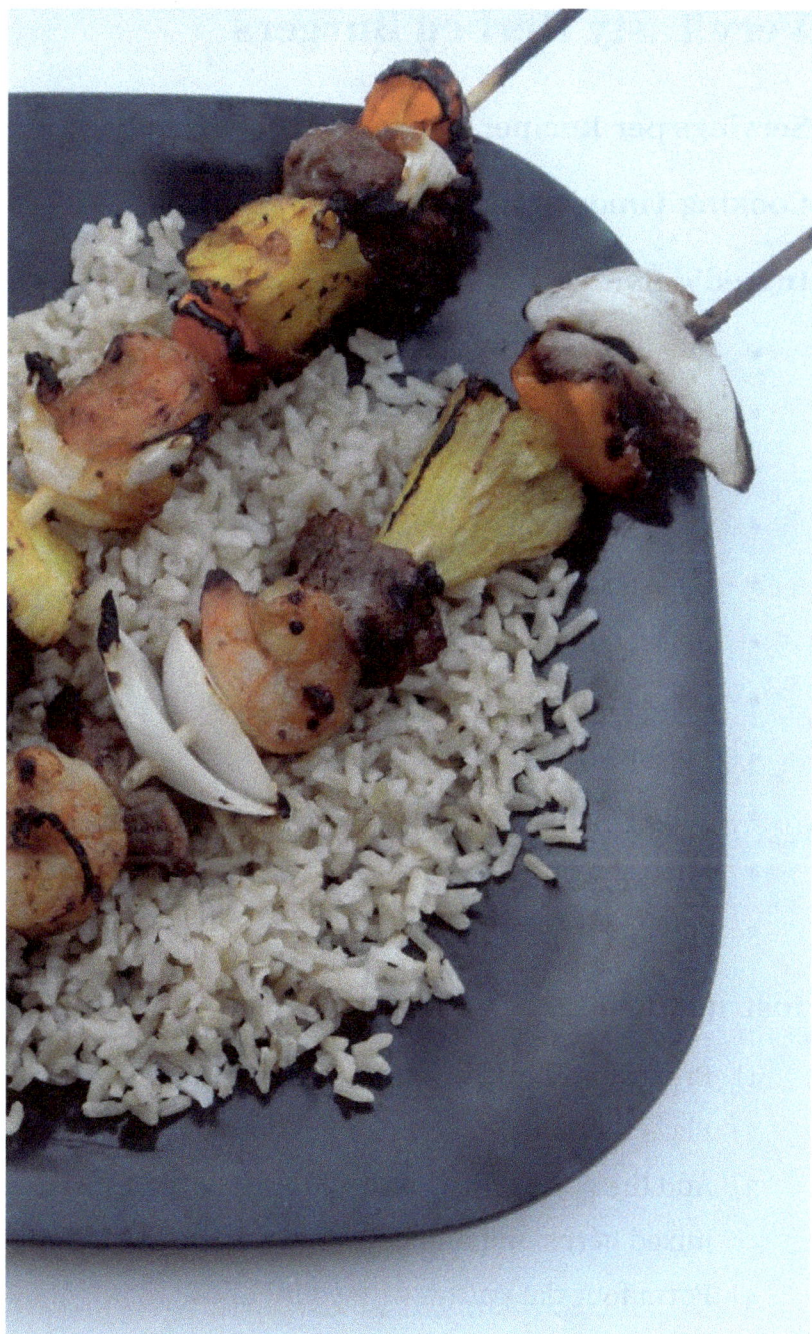

Very Tasty Herbed Burgers

Servings per Recipe: 4

Cooking Time: 25 minutes

Ingredients:

- ¼ cup grated cheddar cheese /32.5G
- ½ pound minced pork or beef /225G
- 1 onion, chopped
- 1 tablespoon basil /15G
- 1 teaspoon minced garlic /5G
- 1 teaspoon mixed herbs /5G
- 1 teaspoon mustard /5G
- 1 teaspoon tomato puree /5G
- 4 bread buns
- Mixed greens
- Salt and pepper to taste

Instructions:

1) Preheat mid-air fryer to 390° F or 199°C .
2) Place the grill pan accessory in the air fryer.
3) Add the pork, onion, garlic, tomato puree, mustard, basil, mixed herbs, salt and pepper in a mixing bowl. Mix well.
4) Form four flat patties with your hands.
5) Place on the grill pan accessory.

6) Cook for 25 minutes. Flip the burgers regularly throughout the cooking process.

7) Serve patties on bread buns and dress with cheese and mixed greens.

Nutrition information:

- Calories per serving: 548
- Carbs: 24.4g
- Protein: 16.1g
- Fat: 42.8g

Air Fried Chicken Tenderloin

Serves: 8

Cooking Time: 15

Ingredients:

- ½ cup almond flour /65G
- 1 egg, beaten
- 2 tablespoons coconut oil /30ML
- 8 chicken tenderloins
- Salt and pepper to taste

Instructions:

1) Preheat the air fryer for 5 minutes.
2) Season the 8 chicken tenderloin with salt and pepper to taste.
3) Dip in beaten eggs then press the chicken sides lightly in almond flour.
4) Place in the air fryer and brush with coconut oil.
5) Cook for 15 minutes at 375O F or 191°C .
6) Shake the air fryer basket after 8 minutes of cooking to give even smoking.

Nutrition information:

- Calories per serving: 130.3
- Carbohydrates: 0.7g

- Protein:8.7 g
- Fat:10.3 g

Almond Flour Battered Chicken Cordon Bleu

Serves: 1

Cooking Time: 30 minutes

Ingredients:

- ¼ cup almond flour /32.5G
- 1 slice cheddar cheese
- 1 slice of ham
- 1 small egg, beaten
- 1 teaspoon parsley /5G
- 2 chicken breasts, butterflied
- Salt and pepper to taste

Instructions:

1) Season the chicken with parsley, salt and pepper to taste.
2) Place the cheese and ham in the middle of the chicken and roll. Secure with a toothpick.
3) Dip the rolled-up chicken in egg and lightly press the sides of the chicken in almond flour.
4) Place in the air fryer.
5) Cook for 30 Minutes at 350° F or 177°C .

Nutrition information:

- Calories per serving: 1142

- Carbohydrates: 5.5g
- Protein: 79.4g
- Fat: 89.1g

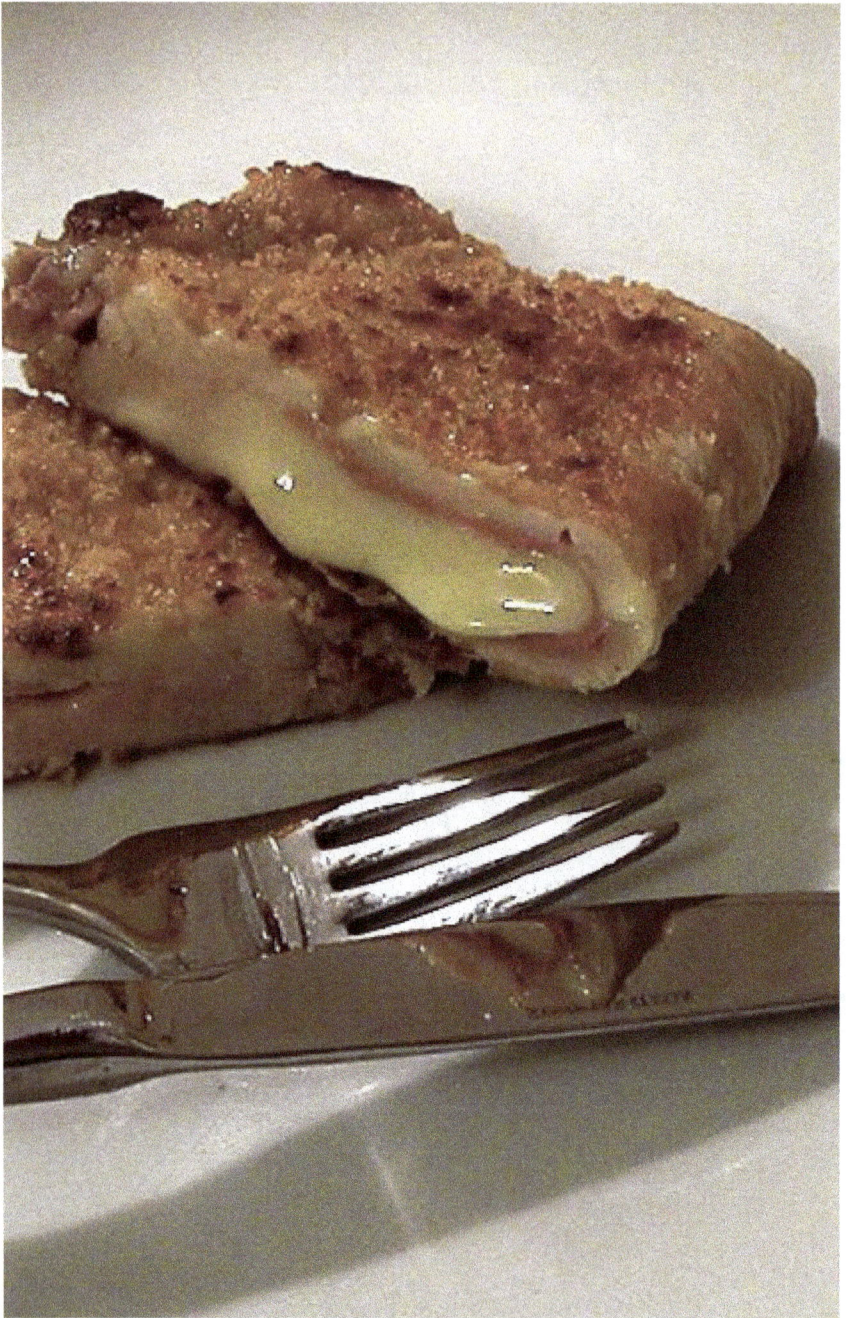

Copycat KFC Chicken Strips

Serves: 8

Cooking Time: 20 Minutes

Ingredients:

- 1 chicken, cut into strips
- 1 egg, beaten
- 2 tablespoons almond flour /30G
- 2 tablespoons desiccated coconut /30G
- A dash of oregano
- A dash of paprika
- A dash of thyme
- Salt and pepper to taste

Instructions:

1) Soak the chicken in egg.
2) Add other ingredients to a mixing bowl and mix properly.
3) Dredge the chicken inside dry ingredients.
4) Place inside the air fryer basket.
5) Cook for 20 Minutes at 350° F or 177°C .

Nutrition information:

- Calories per serving: 100
- Carbohydrates: 0.9g
- Protein: 4.8g

- Fat: 8.6g

Creamy Chicken 'n Pasta Tetrazzini

Servings per Recipe: 3

Cooking Time: 30 Minutes

Ingredients:

- 1 cup chopped cooked chicken /130G
- 1/2 (10.75 ounces) can condensed cream of mushroom soup /322.5ML
- 1/2 cup chicken broth /125ML
- 1/2 cup shredded sharp Cheddar cheese /65G
- 1/4 (10 ounces) package frozen green peas /300G
- 1/4 cup grated Parmesan cheese /32.5G
- 1/4 cup minced green bell pepper 32.5G
- 1/4 cup minced onion 32.5G
- 1/4 teaspoon salt /1.25G
- 1/4 teaspoon Worcestershire sauce /1.25ML
- 1/8 teaspoon ground black pepper /0.625G
- 2 tablespoons butter /30G
- 2 tablespoons cooking sherry /30ML
- 3/4 cup sliced fresh mushrooms /98G
- 4-ounce linguine pasta, cooked following manufacturer's instructions /120G

Instructions:

1) Lightly grease baking pan of air fryer and melt butter for 2 minutes at 360° or 183°C . Stir in bell pepper, onion, and mushrooms. Cook for 5 minutes.

2) Add chicken broth and mushroom soup, mix well. Cook for 5 minutes.

3) Mix in chicken, pepper, salt, Worcestershire sauce, sherry, peas, cheddar cheese, and pasta. Sprinkle paprika and Parmesan at the top.

4) Cook for 15 minutes at 390° F or 199°C until the tops are lightly browned.

5) Serve and enjoy.

Nutrition Information:

- Calories per Serving: 494
- Carbs: 39.0g
- Protein: 28.8g
- Fat: 24.7g

Creamy Chicken 'n Rice

Servings per Recipe: 3

Cooking Time: 45 minutes

Ingredients:

- 1 (10.75 ounces) can cream of celery soup /322.5ML
- 1 (10.75 ounces) can cream of chicken soup /322.5ML
- 1 (10.75 ounces) can cream of mushroom soup /322.5ML
- 1/2 cup butter, sliced into pats /65G
- 2 cups instant white rice /260G
- 2 cups water /500ML
- 3 chicken breasts, cut into cubes
- salt and ground black pepper to taste

Instructions:

1) Grease the baking pan of the air fryer with any oil of your choice using a cooking spray.
2) Mix cream of mushroom, celery soup, chicken soup, rice, water and chicken in a pan. Mix well.
3) Season with pepper and salt. Top with butter pats.
4) Cover the pan with foil, air fry at 360° F or 183°C for 25 minutes.
5) Let it sit for 10 minutes.
6) Serve and enjoy.

Nutrition Information:

- Calories per Serving: 439
- Carbs: 36.7g
- Protein: 16.8g
- Fat: 25.0g

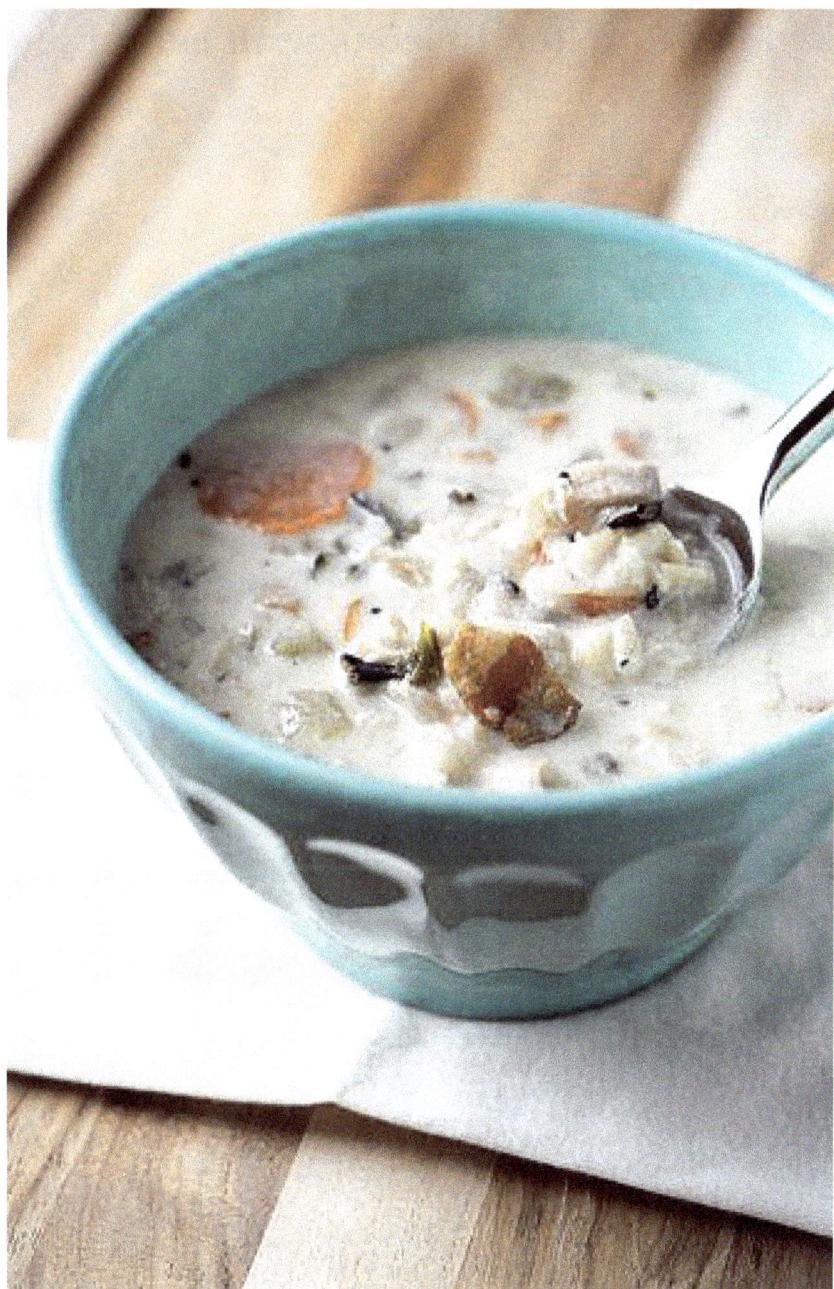

Creamy Chicken Breasts with crumbled Bacon

Serves: 4

Cooking Time: 25 minutes

Ingredients:

- ¼ cup essential olive oil /62.5ML
- 1 block cream cheese
- 4 chicken breasts
- 8 slices of bacon, fried and crumbled
- Salt and pepper to taste

Instructions:

1) Preheat mid-air fryer for 5 minutes.
2) Place the chicken breasts in a baking pan.
3) Add the essential olive oil and cream cheese. Season with salt and pepper to taste.
4) Place the baking dish and cook for 25 minutes at 350° F or 177°C .
5) Sprinkle crumbled bacon after air frying.

Nutrition information:

- Calories per serving: 827
- Carbohydrates: 1.7g
- Protein: 61.2g

- Fat: 67.9g

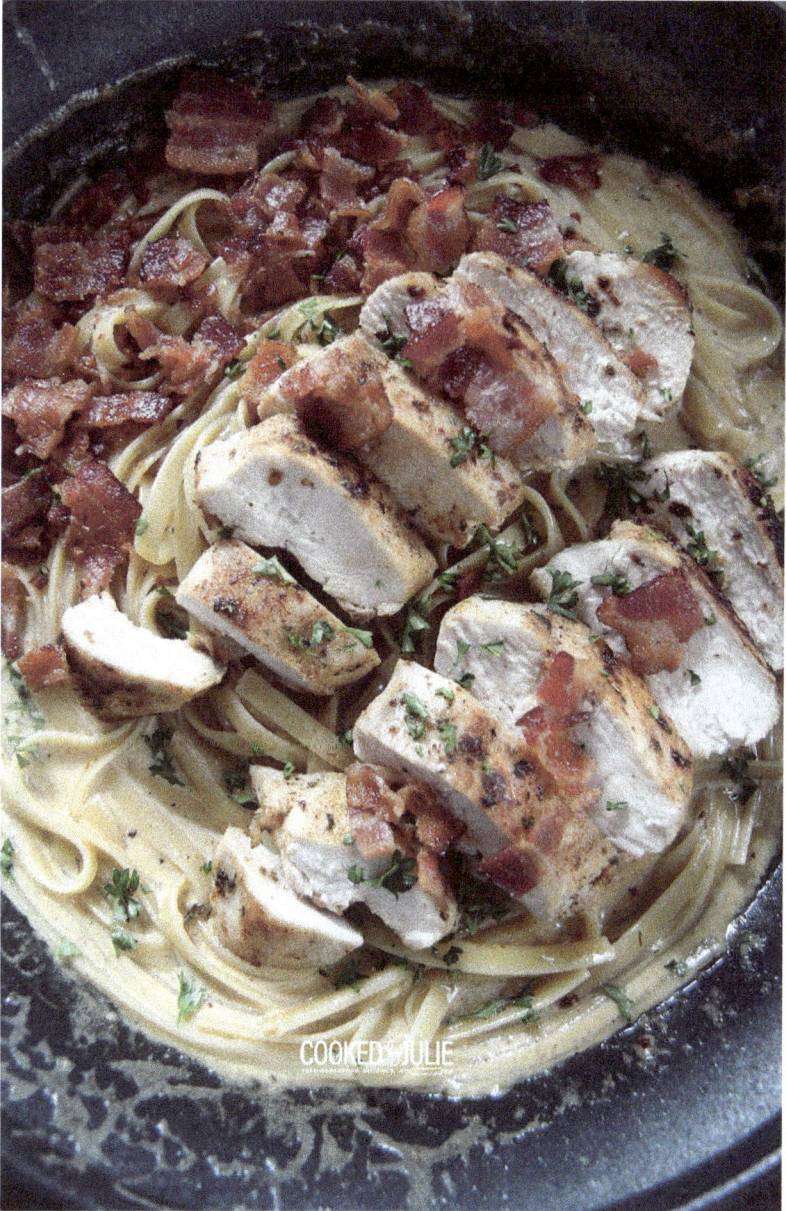

Creamy Chicken-Veggie Pasta

Servings per Recipe: 3

Cooking Time: 30 Minutes

Ingredients:

- 3 chicken tenderloins, cut into chunks
- salt and pepper to taste
- garlic powder to taste
- 1 cup frozen mixed vegetables /130G
- 1 tablespoon grated Parmesan cheese /15G
- 1 tablespoon butter, melted /15ML
- 1/2 (10.75 ounces) can condensed cream of chicken soup /322.5ML
- 1/2 (10.75 ounces) can condensed cream of mushroom soup 322.5ML
- 1/2 cup dry fusilli pasta, cooked based on manufacturer's Instructions/65G
- 1 tablespoon and 1-1/2 teaspoons essential olive oil /22.5ML
- 1-1/2 teaspoons dried minced onion /7.5G
- 1-1/2 teaspoons dried basil /7.5G
- 1-1/2 teaspoons dried parsley /7.5G
- 1/2 cup dry bread crumbs /65G

Instructions:

1) Grease the baking pan of the air fryer with oil. Add chicken and season with parsley, basil, garlic powder, pepper, salt, and minced onion. For 10 minutes, cook at 360° F or 183°C , stir halfway through cooking time.

2) Stir in mixed vegetables, mushroom soup, chicken soup, and cooked pasta. Mix well.

3) Mix well butter, Parmesan cheese, and bread crumbs in a small bowl and spread on top of casserole.

4) Cook for 20 minutes or until tops are lightly browned.

5) Serve and enjoy.

Nutrition Information:

- Calories per Serving: 399
- Carbs: 35.4g
- Protein: 19.8g
- Fat: 19.8g

Meat-Covered Boiled Eggs

Serves: 7

Cooking Time: 25 minutes

Ingredients:

¼ cup coconut flour /32.5G

1-pound ground beef /450G

2 eggs, beaten

2 tablespoons butter, melted /30ML

7 large eggs, boiled and peeled

Cooking spray

Salt and pepper to taste

Instructions:

1) Preheat mid-air fryer for 5 minutes.
2) Place the beaten eggs, ground beef, butter, and coconut flour in a mixing bowl. Season with salt and pepper to taste.
3) Coat the boiled eggs with all the meat mixture, place in the fridge to set for 120 minutes.
4) Grease the baking pan with cooking spray.
5) Place inside the air fryer basket.
6) Cook at 350° F or 177°C for 25 minutes.

Nutrition information:

- Calories per serving: 325
- Carbohydrates: 1.8g
- Protein: 21.4g
- Fat: 25.8g

Middle Eastern Chicken BBQ with Tzatziki Sauce

Servings per Recipe: 6

Cooking Time: 24 minutes

Ingredients:

- 1 1/2 pounds skinless, boneless chicken halves - cut into bite-sized pieces /675G
- 1 teaspoon dried oregano /5G
- 1/2 teaspoon salt /2.5G
- 1/4 cup essential olive oil /62.5ML
- 2 cloves garlic, minced
- 2 tablespoons lemon juice /30ML

- Tzatziki Dip Ingredients

- 1 (6 ounces) container plain Greek-style yogurt /180ML
- 1 tablespoon extra virgin olive oil /15ML
- 2 teaspoons white wine vinegar /10ML
- 1 clove garlic, minced
- 1 pinch of salt
- 1/2 cucumber - peeled, seeded, and grated

Instructions:

1) Mix all the Tzatziki dip Ingredients in a medium-sized bowl. Refrigerate for at least 120 minutes.

2) Mix salt, oregano, garlic, lemon juice, and organic olive oil in a bowl. Mix well. Add chicken, squeeze excess air, seal, and marinate for at least some hours.

3) Thread chicken into skewers and put on a skewer rack. Cook in batches.

4) For 12 minutes, cook on 360° F or 183°C . Halfway through cooking time, turnover skewers and baste with marinade.

5) Serve and enjoy with Tzatziki dip.

Nutrition Information:

- Calories per Serving: 264
- Carbs: 2.6g
- Protein: 25.5g
- Fat: 16.8g

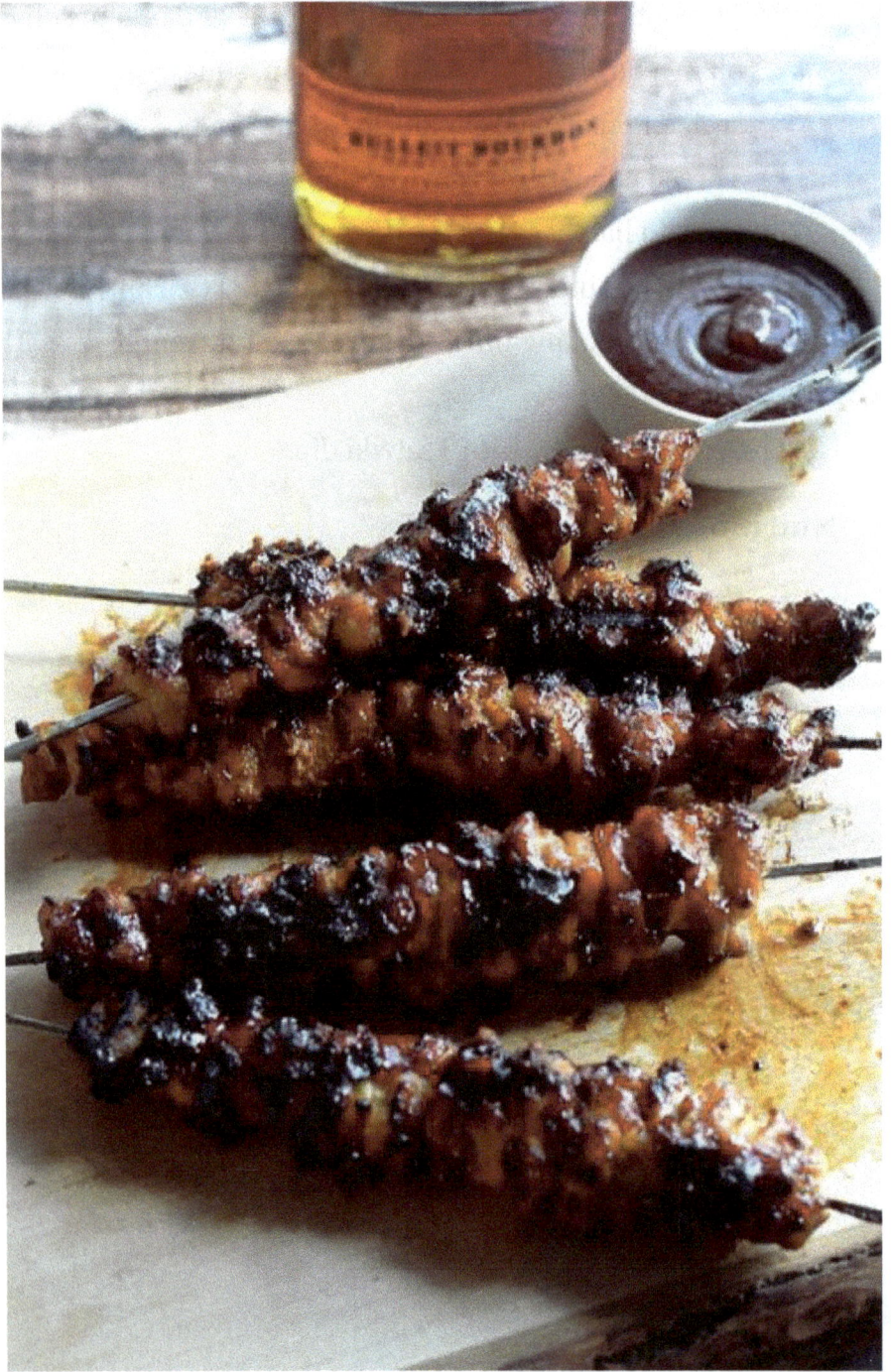

Mixed Vegetable Breakfast Frittata

Servings per Recipe: 6

Cooking Time: 45 minutes

Ingredients:

- ½-pound breakfast sausage /225G
- 1 cup cheddar cheese shredded /130G
- 1 teaspoon kosher salt /5G
- 1/2 cup milk or cream /125ML
- 1/2 teaspoon black pepper /2.5G
- 6 eggs
- 8-ounces frozen mixed vegetables (sweet peppers, broccoli, etc.), thawed /240G

Instructions:

1) Oil baking pan lightly with cooking spray. Cook the breakfast sausage at 360° F or 183°C for 10 minutes crush the sausage until you get ground meat. After 5 minutes crush again. Remove excess fat when cooing is done.

2) Stir in thawed mixed vegetables and cook for 7 minutes or until heated through, stirring halfway through cooking time.

3) Whisk eggs, cream, salt, and pepper well in a bowl.

4) Evenly spread the vegetable mixture in the air fryer basket and pour in the egg mixture. Cover pan with foil.

5) Cook for 15 minutes, remove foil and continue cooking for additional 5-10 minutes or until eggs are well cooked.

6) Serve and enjoy.

Nutrition Information:

- Calories per Serving: 187
- Carbs: 7.0g
- Protein: 15.0g
- Fat: 11.0g

Mushroom 'n Coconut Cream Quiche

Serves: 8

Cooking Time: 20 minutes

Ingredients:

- ¼ cup coconut cream /62.5ML
- ½ cup almond flour /65G
- ½ cup mushroom, sliced /65G
- ½ onion, chopped
- 1 tablespoon chives, chopped /15G
- 2 tablespoons coconut oil /30ML
- 4 eggs, beaten
- Salt and pepper to taste

Instructions:

1) Preheat the air fryer for 5 minutes.
2) Add the almond flour and coconut oil.
3) Put the almond flour mixture at the bottom of the baking dish.
4) Place inside air fryer and cook for 5 minutes.
5) Meanwhile, add other ingredients to the mixing bowl. Mix well.
6) Take the crust out and pour over the egg mixture.
7) Put the baking dish back into the air fryer and cook for 15 minutes at 350° F or 177°C .

Nutrition information:

- Calories per serving: 125
- Carbohydrates: 2.2g
- Protein: 4.8g
- Fat: 10.8g

Coconutty Lemon Bars

Serves: 12

Cooking Time: 25 minutes

Ingredients:

- ¼ cup cashew /32.5G
- ¼ cup fresh lemon juice, freshly squeezed /62.5ML
- ¾ cup coconut milk /188ML
- ¾ cup erythritol /98G
- 1 cup desiccated coconut /130G
- 1 teaspoon baking powder /5G
- 2 eggs, beaten
- 2 tablespoons coconut oil /30ML
- A dash of salt

Instructions

1) Preheat the air fryer for 5 minutes.
2) Combine all ingredients and mix well.
3) Use a hand mixer to blend everything.
4) Pour into a baking dish.
5) Bake for 25 minutes at 350° F or 177°C or until a toothpick inserted in middle comes clean.

Nutrition information:

- Calories per serving: 118

- Carbohydrates: 3.9g
- Protein: 2.6g
- Fat:10.2g

Coffee 'n Blueberry Cake

Servings per Recipe: 6

Cooking Time: 35 minutes

Ingredients:

- 1 cup white sugar /130G
- 1 egg
- 1/2 cup butter, softened /65G
- 1/2 cup fresh or frozen blueberries /65G
- 1/2 cup sour cream /125ML
- 1/2 teaspoon baking powder /2.5G
- 1/2 teaspoon ground cinnamon /2.5G
- 1/2 teaspoon vanilla flavoring /2.5G
- 1/4 cup brown sugar /32.5G
- 1/4 cup chopped pecans /32.5G
- 1/8 teaspoon salt /0.625G
- 1-1/2 teaspoons confectioners' sugar for dusting /7.5G
- 3/4 cup and 1 tablespoon all-purpose flour /112.5G

Instructions:

1) Mix pecans, cinnamon, and brown sugar.
2) Blend all wet ingredients. Add dry ingredients except confectioner's sugar and blueberries. Blend well until smooth and creamy.
3) Grease baking pan with oil.

4) Pour half of the batter into the pan. Sprinkle ½ of pecan mixture on top. Pour the remaining batter. And top with the remaining pecan mixture.

5) Cover pan with foil.

6) Cook for 35 minutes at 330° F or 166°C .

7) Serve with a dusting of confectioner's sugar and enjoy.

Nutrition Information:

- Calories per Serving: 471
- Carbs: 59.5g
- Protein: 4.1g
- Fat: 24.0g

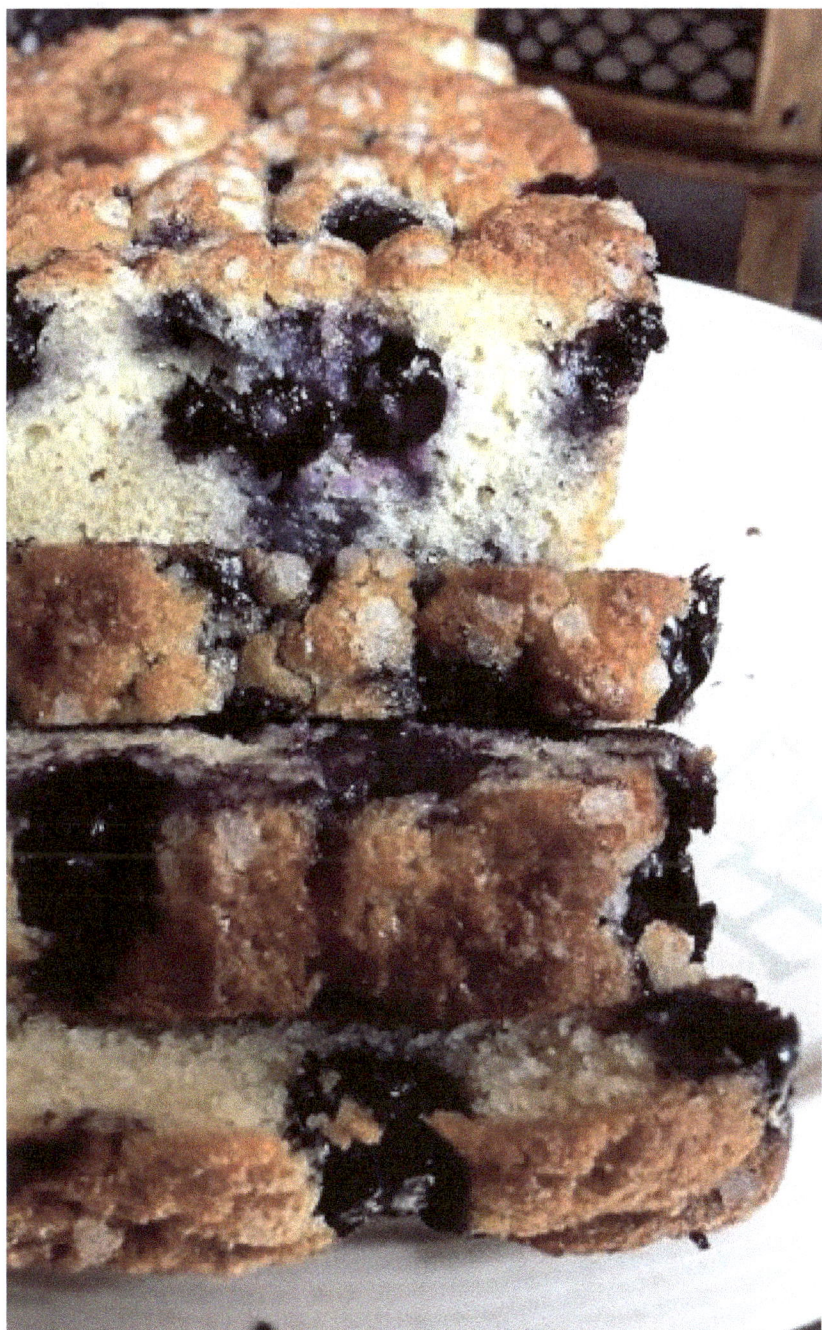

Coffee Flavored Cookie Dough

Serves: 12

Cooking Time: 20 Minutes

Ingredients:

- ¼ cup butter /32.5G
- ¼ teaspoon xanthan gum /1.25G
- ½ teaspoon coffee espresso powder /2.5G
- ½ teaspoon stevia powder /2.5G
- ¾ cup almond flour /98G
- 1 egg
- 1 teaspoon vanilla /5G
- 1/3 cup sesame seeds /43G
- 2 tablespoons cocoa powder /30G
- 2 tablespoons cream cheese, softened /30G

Instructions:

1) Preheat the air fryer for 5 minutes.
2) Combine all ingredients inside a mixing bowl.
3) Press right into a baking dish that can fit in the air fryer.
4) Place in mid-air fryer basket and cook for 20 minutes at 400° F or 205°C or if a toothpick inserted inside come out clean.

Nutrition information:

- Calories per serving: 88
- Carbohydrates: 1.3g
- Protein: 1.9g
- Fat: 8.3g

Coffee Flavored Doughnuts

Serves: 6

Cooking Time: 6 minutes

Ingredients:

- ¼ cup coconut sugar /32.5G
- ¼ cup coffee /32.5G
- ½ teaspoon salt /2.5G
- 1 cup white all-purpose flour /130G
- 1 tablespoon sunflower oil /15ML
- 1 teaspoon baking powder /5G
- 2 tablespoon aquafaba /30ML

Instructions:

1) Mix the dry ingredients flour, sugar, salt, and baking powder.
2) Mix the aquafaba, sunflower oil, and coffee.
3) Mix to make a dough.
4) Allow the dough to sit in the fridge.
5) Preheat air fryer to 400° F or 205°C .
6) Knead the dough and form doughnuts.
7) Place in a single layer in the air fryer and cook for 6 minutes.
8) Avoid shaking the pan to keep the donut in shape.

Nutrition information:

- Calories per serving: 113
- Carbohydrates: 20.45g
- Protein: 2.16g
- Fat:2.54g

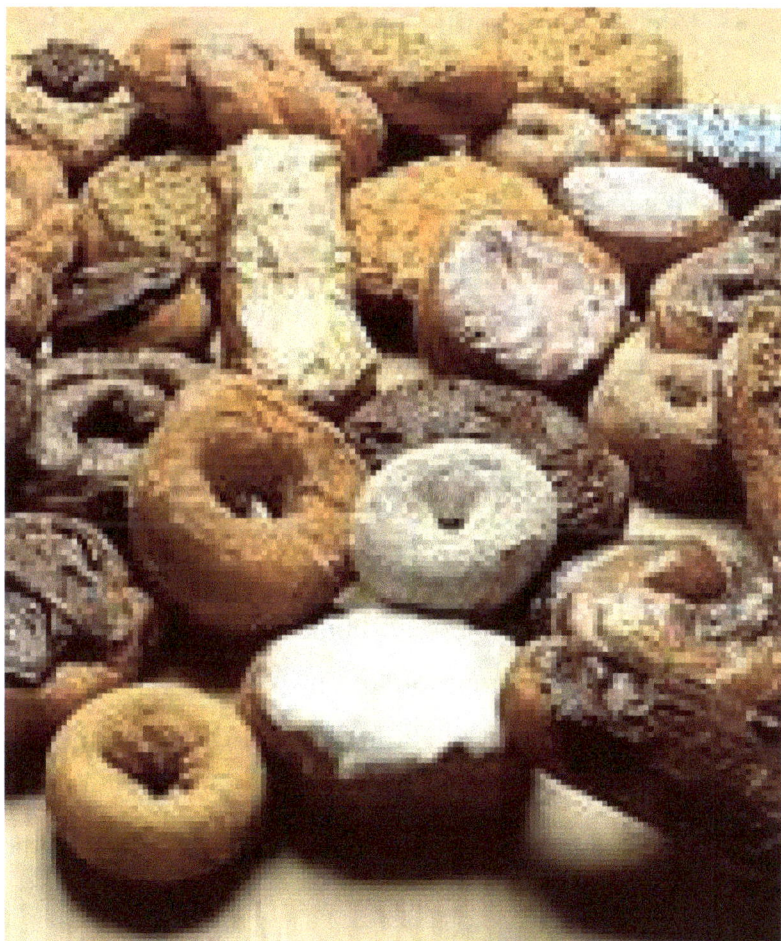

Crisped 'n Chewy Chonut Holes

Serves: 6

Cooking Time: 10 minutes

Ingredients:

- ¼ cup almond milk /62.5ML
- ¼ cup coconut sugar /32.5G
- ¼ teaspoon cinnamon /1.25G
- ½ teaspoon salt /2.5G
- 1 cup white all-purpose flour /130G
- 1 tablespoon coconut oil, melted /15ML
- 1 teaspoon baking powder /5G
- 2 tablespoon aquafaba or liquid from canned chickpeas /30ML

Instructions:

1) Mix the flour, sugar, and baking powder in a bowl. Add the salt and cinnamon and mix well.
2) Mix the coconut oil, aquafaba, and almond milk in another bowl.
3) Gently pour the dry ingredients on the wet ingredients. Mix until well combined.
4) Place the dough inside a refrigerator to rest for about an hour.
5) Preheat mid-air fryer to 370° F or 191°C .

6) Make small balls with the dough and set them inside the air fryer and cook for 10 minutes. Do not shake the air fryer.
7) Once cooked, sprinkle with sugar and cinnamon.
8) Serve with your breakfast coffee.

Nutrition information:

- Calories per serving: 120
- Carbohydrates: 21.62g
- Protein: 2.31g
- Fat:2.76g